# Using This Manual

This manual is designed to be very straight forward and easy to use.

Review this manual before beginning the U-ExCEL Balancing Act program, it is important to be familiar with the various instructions. This manual is organized to: (1) introduce you to the U-ExCEL Balancing Act Program, (2) offer step by step instructions to perform and practice a variety of balance specific exercises in order to maintain or improve balance and stability, and (3) check performance at the end of the Beginner, Intermediate, and Advanced level exercises.

For those with visual impairments, The Iris Network, in Portland Maine and the State of Maine's Division for the Blind and Visually Impaired have assisted to create a large print and abridged version of this manual, which includes only the exercises. Contact us if you would like to order the abridged large print version of the U-ExCEL Balancing Act Manual.

## Individual Use

This manual is designed for individuals to take home and use independently. We recommend that you start with the beginner level exercises and progress as you feel comfortable.

## Health Providers and Group Use

If you are a part of a group and wish to use this program see **Appendix D**: Key Points for Health Providers and Community Organizations.

# Balancing Act Participant Instructions

## a) Getting Started

You can begin the exercises within this manual at any time. Instructions for how to perform each exercise are listed in the Balancing Act Exercises section (beginning on page 4). There are few general instructions:

- Balance exercises should be done in front of a stable surface you can hold on to if needed (i.e. hand rail, counter, heavy chair, or table)
- Start with the beginner exercises, regardless of balance ability
- Review the hand positions, and start with Hand Position #1. Reduce contact to Hand Position #3 as you feel more confident
- Hold each exercise for <u>5 seconds</u> and build up to <u>30 seconds</u>
- It is normal for your body to move (sway, or shake) when doing balance exercises – this is your body learning to balance
  - ➤ If you aren't comfortable with this movement bring hands to the stable surface to regain balance
- At first all exercises should be performed with eyes open, for 30 seconds and Hand Position #3. Too easy? Try closing your eyes during each exercise. When you close your eyes, start with Hand Position #1 or #2 before you progress to Hand Position #3
- Progressing through the exercises takes time and advancing to the next level of exercises should only be done when stability is attained for 30 seconds using Hand Position #3
  - ➤ Be sure you are able to complete the "STOP" Checklist before advancing to the next level of exercises. The "STOP" page is at the end of each exercise level
- The fastest way to improve balance is to do 5 Balancing Act exercises **every day**, practicing each exercise 3 times. Too much? Do them at least 3 days a week.
- Balancing Act exercises can be done any time during the day and need not be done all at once
  - ➤ They can be practiced during commercials while watching television or when near a table or stable surface. They can be done while waiting in the grocery line, or while doing chores such as cooking, ironing or getting dressed

**NOTE: Know your own limitations!**
If at any time you feel dizzy or short of breath, stop exercising and contact your physician.

## b) Keeping Track of U-ExCEL Balancing Act Training

U-ExCEL Balancing Act works best when participants track their progress over time. Some helpful tips and tools for keeping track of your balance exercise program are provided in **Appendix A**.

## c) Importance of Having a Support System

U-ExCEL Balancing Act works best when you identify a person who will check in with you on a regular basis to ask if you are doing your exercises. Doing the exercises is the key to improving balance and being reminded helps! See **Appendix B** and fill in the **Social Support Identifier** to identify the best person to provide support.

## d) Hand Positions

The hands are very useful in balance training, especially when first beginning to do Balancing Act exercises or when trying a more difficult balance exercise.

**Hand Position #1**: Both hands hold onto a stable surface. Provides the most stability with the greatest point of contact (**Appendix E**) with the stable surface.

**Hand Position #2**: Finger tips of both hands rest on a stable surface. Provides some stability and has less point of contact with the stable surface while making it easy to hold on with both hands if there is too much *postural sway* (see Glossary in **Appendix E**).

**Hand Position #3**: Both hands hover a few inches above a stable surface. Provides no point of contact from hands, so the body works to stay balanced. This hand position still makes it easy to grab on to a stable surface if needed.

| #1 | #2 | #3 |
|----|----|----|

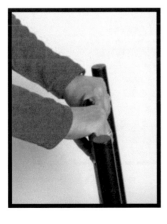 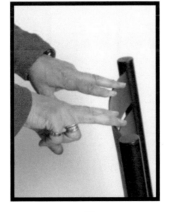 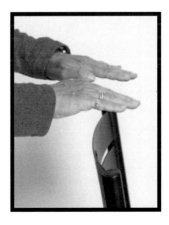

# Balancing Act: Beginner Exercises

**Instructions for all exercises:**
- Hold each position for 5 seconds, building up to 30 seconds
- Progress through hand positions (see page 3) with a goal of not holding on – Hand Position #3
- Do exercises #1-#5 and then repeat these two more times
- Too Easy? Perform with eyes closed (only if you feel comfortable)
- It is okay to rest

**Hand Positions reminder:**
- #1.   Holding on with both hands
- #2.   Fingers resting on stable surface
- #3.   Hands hovering above stable surface

**Start Position for all exercises:**
- Stand facing the stable object
- Hands holding on – or ready to hold on
- Stand with back straight, in line with shoulders, knees relaxed
- Feet at comfortable stance
- Weight even on both feet

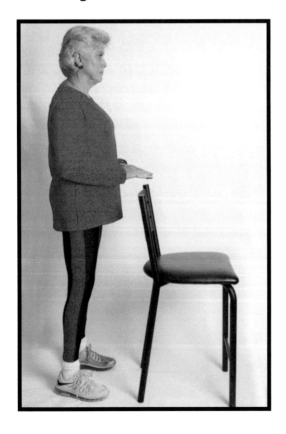 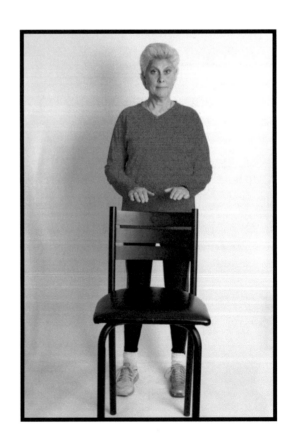

# 1. Feet Shoulder Width

- Stand in Start Position
- Bring feet shoulder width apart, about 12 inches
- Weight even on both feet
- Hold position

Too Easy?
- Don't hold on
- Close your eyes

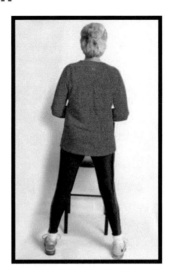

# 2. Feet Hip Width

- Stand in Start Position
- Bring feet hip width apart, about 6 inches
- Weight even on both feet
- Hold position

Too Easy?
- Don't hold on
- Close your eyes

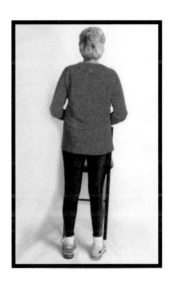

# 3. Feet Together

- Stand in Start Position
- Bring feet close together
- Weight even on both feet
- Hold position

Too Easy?
- Don't hold on
- Close your eyes

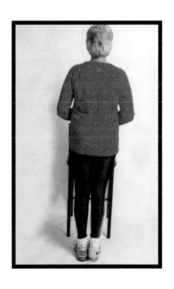

## 4. Foot Forward (feet flat)

- Stand in Start Position
- Step forward with right foot, keeping feet flat
- Weight even on both feet
- Hold position
- Switch and repeat with left foot

Too Easy?
- Don't hold on
- Close your eyes

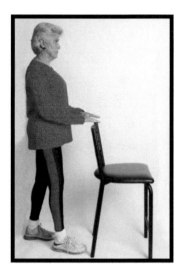

## 5. Weight Shift

- Stand in Start Position
- Bring feet shoulder width apart, about 12 inches
- Shift weight to right side, keep both feet flat
- Keep shoulders and hips in line
- Hold position
- Switch and repeat on the left side

Too Easy?
- Don't hold on
- Close your eyes

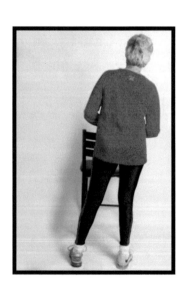

# Stop!

*Before moving on to the next level of balancing exercises, be sure you can answer yes to the following statements for all of the exercises in the beginner level:*

☑ **I can confidently perform the beginner exercises**

☑ **I can perform the beginner exercises for 30 seconds**

☑ **I can perform the beginner exercises without holding on**

# Balancing Act: Intermediate Exercises

**Instructions for all exercises:**
- Hold each position for 5 seconds, building up to 30 seconds
- Progress through hand positions (see page 3) with a goal of not holding on – Hand Position #3
- Do exercises #6-#10 and then repeat these two more times
- Too Easy? Perform with eyes closed (only if you feel comfortable)
- It is okay to rest

**Hand Positions reminder:**
- #1. Holding on with both hands
- #2. Fingers resting on stable surface
- #3. Hands hovering above stable surface

**Start Position for all exercises:**
- Stand facing the stable object
- Hands holding on – or ready to hold on
- Stand with back straight, in line with shoulders, knees relaxed
- Feet at comfortable stance
- Weight even on both feet

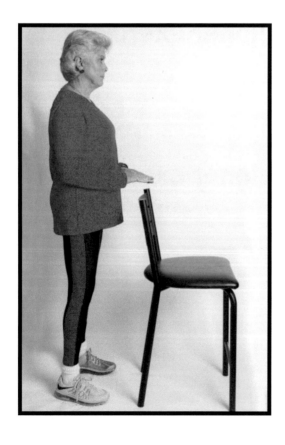
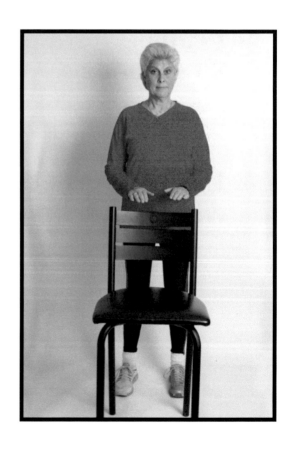

# 6. Feet Together

- Stand in Start Position
- Bring feet close together
- Weight even on both feet
- Hold position

Too Easy?
- Don't hold on
- Close your eyes

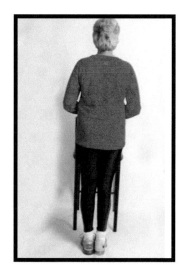

# 7. Heel Forward

- Stand in Start Position
- Step forward with right foot, heel on the ground and toes up
- Left foot remains flat
- Weight even on both feet
- Hold position
- Switch and repeat stepping forward with left foot

Too Easy?
- Don't hold on
- Close your eyes

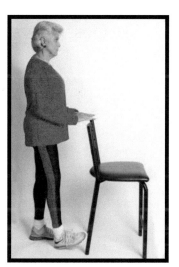

# 8. Toe Back

- Stand in Start Position
- Step back with right foot, toes on the ground and heel up
- Left foot remains flat
- Weight even on both feet
- Hold position
- Switch and repeat stepping back with left foot

Too Easy?
- Don't hold on
- Close your eyes

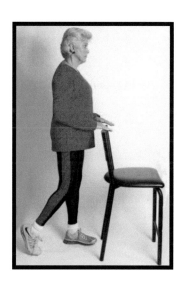

# 9. Heel to Toe (broad stance)

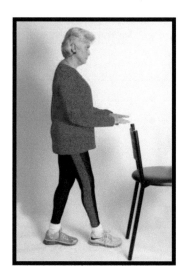

- Stand in Start Position
- Step forward with right foot, placing foot in front of left with 5 inches between heel and toe
- Weight even on both feet
- Hold position
- Switch and repeat with left foot in front

Too Easy?
- Don't hold on
- Close your eyes

# 10. Toe to Side

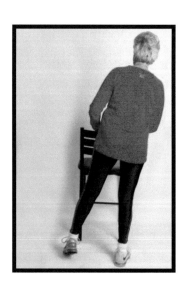

- Stand in Start Position
- Bring feet shoulder width apart, about 12 inches
- Shift weight to right side, going onto left toe as more weight shifts to right side
- Keep shoulders and hips in line
- Hold position
- Switch and repeat on the left side

Too Easy?
- Shift more weight to right foot
- Go higher onto toe
- Don't hold on
- Close your eyes

# Stop!

*Before moving on to the next level of balancing exercises, be sure you can answer yes to the following statements for all of the exercises in the intermediate level:*

☑ **I can confidently perform the intermediate exercises**

☑ **I can perform the intermediate exercises for 30 seconds**

☑ **I can perform the intermediate exercises without holding on**

# Balancing Act: Advanced Exercises

**Instructions for all exercises:**
- Hold each position for 5 seconds, building up to 30 seconds
- Progress through hand positions (see page 3) with a goal of not holding on – Hand Position #3
- Do exercises #11-#15 and then repeat these two more times
- Challenge: perform with eyes closed (only if you feel comfortable)
- It is okay to rest

**Hand Positions reminder:**
- #1.   Holding on with both hands
- #2.   Fingers resting on stable surface
- #3.   Hands hovering above stable surface

**Start Position for all exercises:**
- Stand facing the stable object
- Hands holding on – or ready to hold on
- Stand with back straight, in line with shoulders, knees relaxed
- Feet at comfortable stance
- Weight even on both feet

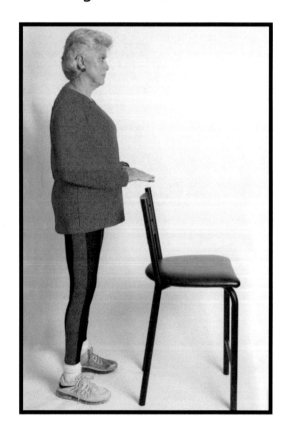 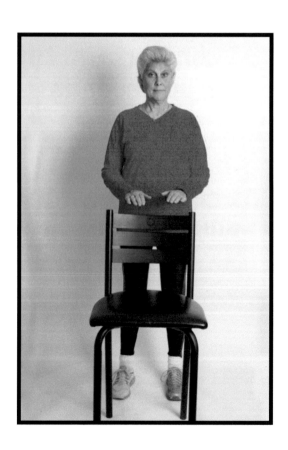

# 11. Heel to Toe (touching)

- Stand in Start Position
- Step forward with right foot, bringing the heel of right foot to the toes of left foot
- Toes of both feet pointing forward
- Weight even on both feet
- Hold position
- Switch and repeat with left foot in front

Too Easy?
- Don't hold on
- Close your eyes

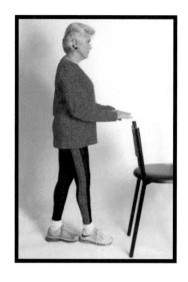

# 12. Weight Shift (foot up)

- Stand in Start Position
- Bring feet shoulder width apart, about 12 inches
- Shift all weight to right side, allowing left foot to come off the ground
- Keep shoulder and hip in line
- Hold position
- Switch and repeat on the left side

Too Easy?
- Lift foot higher off the ground to the side
- Don't hold on
- Close your eyes

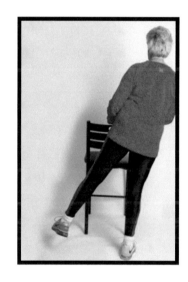

# 13. Foot Forward

- Stand in Start Position
- Step forward with right foot, heel on the ground, toes up
- Left foot remains flat
- Shift weight back to left foot, lift right foot off the ground in front of you
- Hold position
- Switch and repeat stepping forward with left foot

Too Easy?
- Lift foot higher off the ground in front of you
- Don't hold on
- Close your eyes

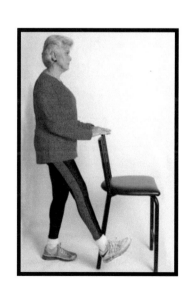

# 14. Foot Back

- Stand in Start Position
- Step back with right foot, toes on the ground and heel up
- Left foot remains flat
- Shift weight forward to left foot, lift right foot off the ground behind you
- Hold position
- Switch and repeat stepping back with left foot

Too Easy?
- Lift foot higher off the ground behind you
- Don't hold on
- Close your eyes

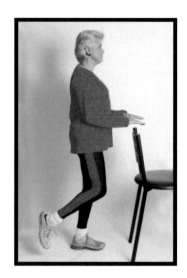

# 15. Knee Up

- Stand in Start Position
- Slowly lift right knee up, as if going into a march
    - Goal is to lift knee up to hip height (Keep knee lower to make easier)
- Hold position
- Switch and repeat bringing left knee up

Too Easy?
- Lift knee up higher
- Don't hold on
- Close your eyes

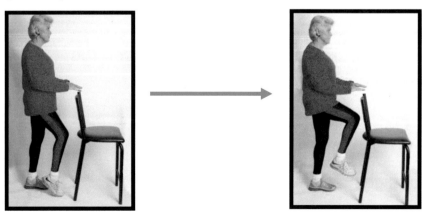

# Stop!

*Before moving on to the next level of balancing exercises, be sure you can answer yes to the following statements for all of the exercises in the advanced level:*

☑ **I can confidently perform the advanced exercises**

☑ **I can perform the advanced exercises for 30 seconds**

☑ **I can perform the advanced exercises without holding on**

# Balancing Act:
## Action Exercises

*Action exercises should only be performed once all advanced exercises can be completed with confidence, without holding on, for 30 seconds.*

### Instructions for Action Exercises:
- These are movement based and should be done only after you have mastered the Advanced Exercises.
- Be sure a stable surface is within reach (i.e. hand rail, wall, chair, etc)
- Do these exercises slowly
  - The slower they are done, the more balance is challenged
- Progress through hand positions with a goal of not holding on – Hand Position #3
- Do each exercise #16-#20, and then repeat two more times

### Hand Positions reminder:
#1. Holding on with one hand
#2. Fingers resting on stable surface
#3. Hand hovering above stable surface

# 16. Sit to Stand

- Sit in a firm chair
- Slide forward as far as possible
- Slide heels back so they are lined up with the front edge of the chair seat
- Keep back straight, feet shoulder width apart and flat on the ground
- Place hands on knees and lean upper body forward (think nose over toes)
- Use buttock and leg muscles to stand up
  - If needed, use arms to assist
- Stand all the way up and hold for 5 seconds
- Slowly lower back down to chair seat – no plopping
- Repeat 10 times

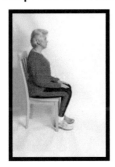 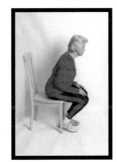 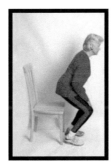 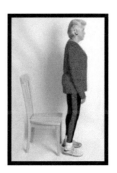

# 17. Arm Swing with Opposite Leg Swing Movement

- Stand in Start Position
- Lift right leg and swing it in front of left leg, at the same time swing left arm behind torso
- Keeping the right foot elevated swing it behind left leg, and swing left arm in front of torso
- Repeat for 10-15 repetitions and then repeat with left leg and right arm

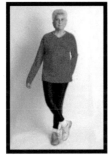 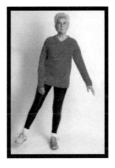 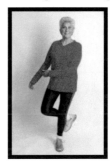

Too Hard?
- Make the arm and leg swing shorter
- Don't cross behind or in front as much

Too Easy?
- Lift leg higher off the ground
- Make swing longer and more exaggerated

# 18. Heel to Toe Walk

- Stand with stable surface to right side, close enough to hold on if needed
- Stand tall, eyes focused in front of you (don't look at feet)
- Raise arms out to the side to aid balance
- Take small step with right foot and place it directly in front of left foot, so the right heel is touching the left toes
- Repeat with left foot
- Continue steps, turn around and return to starting place
- Repeat 3 times down and back

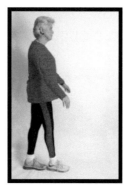 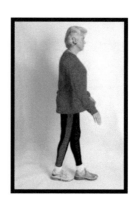

# 19. Exaggerated Walking Steps

- Stand with stable surface to right side, close enough to hold on if needed
- Stand tall, eyes focused in front of you (don't look at feet)
- Raise arms out to the side to aid balance
- Lift right foot off ground, <u>slowly</u> bring foot forward
- Touch right heel to ground, shift weight forward and step on right foot
- Lift left heel and repeat step with left foot
- Continue steps, turn around and return to starting place
- Repeat 3 times down and back

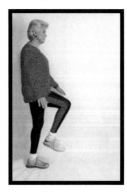 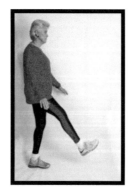 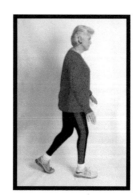 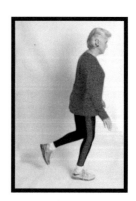

Too Easy?
- Exaggerate each step more by going slower and making the motions bigger – i.e. lift foot higher off the ground, strike with heel, push off with toe

# 20. Grapevine

- Stand facing stable surface, close enough to hold
- Stand tall, eyes focused in front of you (don't look at feet)
- Raise arms out to the side to aid balance
- Moving to the right first, step to side with right foot, and then cross left foot in front of right
- Take another step to side with right foot, and then cross left foot behind right
- Continue this pattern: cross in front, side step, cross behind, and then repeat to the left
- Continue steps, turn around and return to starting place
- Repeat 3 times down and back

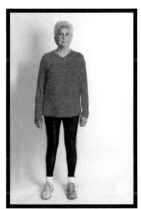 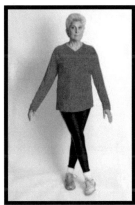 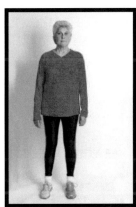 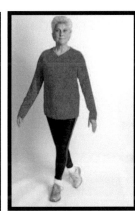 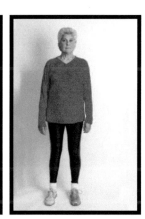

Too Hard?
- Make steps smaller

Too Easy?
- Make bigger steps
- Make sure you're not holding on

# How to Improve Balance

As a Physical Therapist, I've helped thousands of older adults improve balance with exercises, stretches, and balance training programs.

Almost everyone replies YES when I ask them, "Does your balance feel off lately?"

The big question I hear is this: **Can my balance improve?**

The answer is a resounding yes!  Your balance can improve whether you're 45, 65, or 95 years old!

Here are the best ways to improve your balance:

**Exercises-** Exercises for balance that focus on strengthening the muscles in your legs, core, and arms can lead to significant improvements in your balance. There are many exercises to improve balance and 12 that I highly recommend for seniors (see below).

**Stretching -** Improving your flexibility can result in better balance. Stretches can also help improve your posture which can lead to greater stability and improved balance

**Mobility Training -** Joint stiffness can lead to poor mobility, which you've probably noticed at times when you get up and down from a chair. Improving mobility can lead to improved balance and coordination.

If you're curious on the balance research that supports this, you can find the references at the bottom of the PDF.  Nothing like science to back up the importance of balance exercises!

# Single Leg Stance

**Instructions:**

Start with your feet at hip width. While holding onto a counter, lift one foot off the ground slightly. Keep your body tall and avoid leaning onto the planted foot.

Progress this exercise by transitioning to one hand support and eventually no hand support. It's always good to perform near a sturdy counter in case you need to quickly catch your balance.

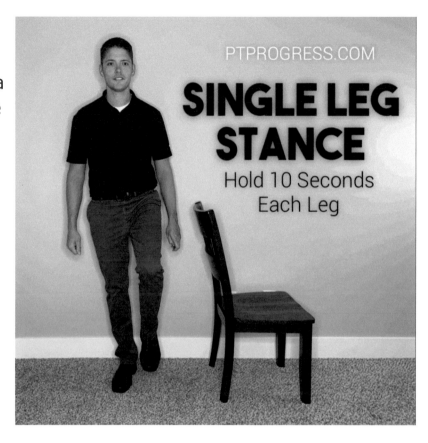

**Hold for 10 to 15 seconds on each leg.**
**Perform 5 times on each leg.**

***Why this is important:*** *This is an essential balance exercise because we stand on one leg every time we take a step or walk up and down stairs! Don't underestimate the importance of the single leg stance exercise!*

# Foot Taps to Step

**Instructions:** *Stand tall facing a step or cone. Beginners should use support from a counter or handrail until your balance improves.*

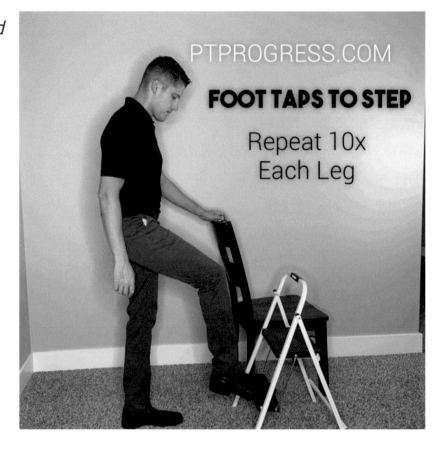

*In a controlled motion, lift one foot and tap the cone or step for one second and return to your starting position. As you repeat this motion, you should focus on consistency and control with each tap.*

**Perform 10 repetitions on each leg.**
**Repeat 2 to 3 times.**

*This exercise is important because it helps with coordination on stairs. How many times have you caught yourself tripping on a step? If you or someone you know has stairs, this is a great balance exercise.*

# Narrow Stance Reaches

**Instructions:** Begin with your feet together or as close as you can while feeling safe. Stand tall and reach forward with one hand while holding onto a counter or solid surface for safety.

Alternate arms as you reach forward. Progress by reaching with both hands forwards.

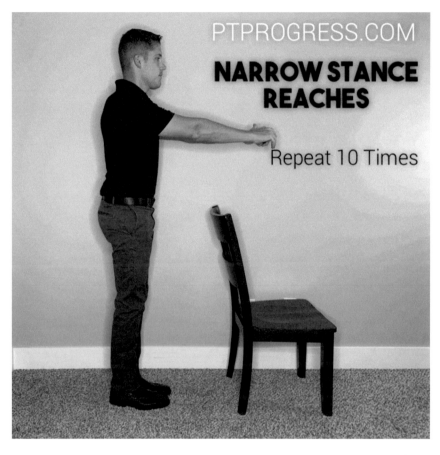

You can make this more challenging by reaching out to the side or in varying directions.

**Perform 10 reaches with each arm.**
**Repeat 2 to 3 times.**

This balance exercise is important because many falls take place while reaching for an item in a tight space.

# 3 Way Hip Kick

**Instructions:** *Stand with your feet shoulder width apart. While holding onto a counter or firm surface, extend your leg forward and return to your starting position.*

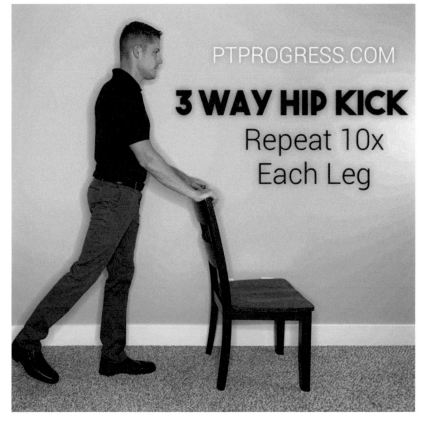

*Repeat this motion to the side returning to the starting position each time. Finally, extend your leg back and return it to the starting position.*

*Perform each motion 5 to 10 times on each leg.*
*Repeat 2 to 3 times.*

*This exercise builds strength in the hip muscles which are important for maintaining stability with walking, turning, and going up and down steps.*

# Standing Marches

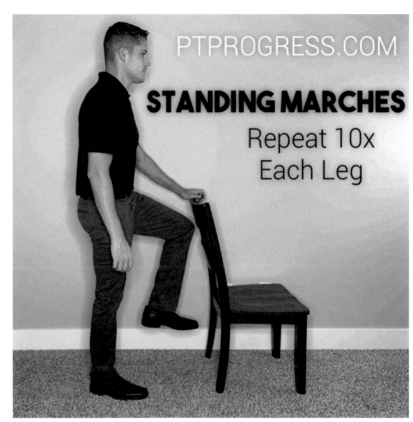

**Instructions:**

*Stand with your feet shoulder width apart. While holding onto a counter or firm surface, raise one leg in a marching motion. Alternate legs and progress difficulty by performing without holding onto the counter or chair.*

*Focus on smooth, controlled movements and keep your body tall to avoid leaning side to side.*

**Perform 20 marches (10 on each leg).**
**Repeat 2 to 3 times.**

*This exercise is great for improving hip strength and single leg balance. If your feet ever catch the ground while you're walking, you'll benefit from this exercise!*

# Mini Lunges

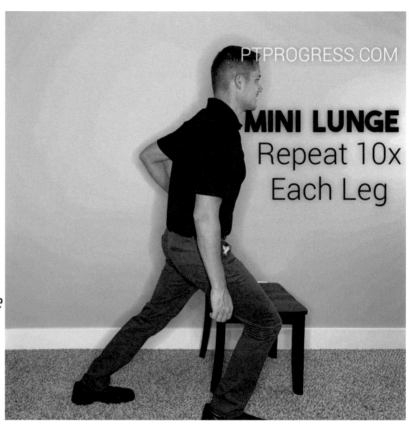

**Instructions:**

Stand with your feet shoulder width apart. While holding onto a counter or firm  surface, step forward  and allow your front  knee to bend slightly.  Return to your starting position and repeat with the  opposite leg.

The lunge does not need to be deep.  If you experience increased knee or hip pain, modify this exercise by  holding onto a counter and taking a smaller step.

**Perform 10 lunges on each leg.**
**Repeat 2 to 3 times.**

This is a helpful balance exercise because it strengthens the legs  while simulating a forward stepping motion.  If you ever feel like  you sometimes stumble forwards, this exercise will help you to  practice catching yourself before you actually fall!

# Lateral Stepping

**Instructions:**

Stand with your feet together. While holding onto a counter or firm surface, step to the side so your feet are just past shoulder width.

Continue this motion along a counter, performing 5 to 10 steps on each side.

**Perform 5 to 10 steps. Repeat 2 to 3 times.**

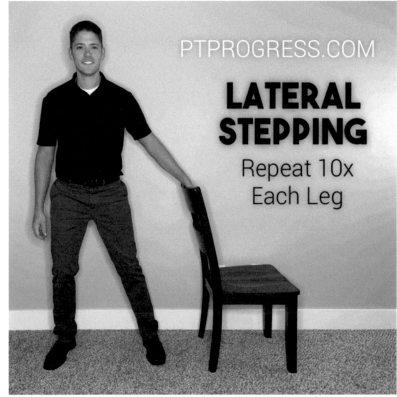

PTPROGRESS.COM

**LATERAL STEPPING**

Repeat 10x
Each Leg

We are constantly turning and sidestepping throughout the day. Unfortunately, this is how many older adults fall. This exercise helps you to become more coordinated with turns and stepping in tight spaces.

# Squats

**Instructions:**

Stand with your feet shoulder width apart.

While holding onto a counter, perform a squatting motion like you are about to sit down.

It can be helpful to position a chair  behind you for safety  and accuracy.

**Perform 10 squats.**
**Repeat 2 to 3 times.**

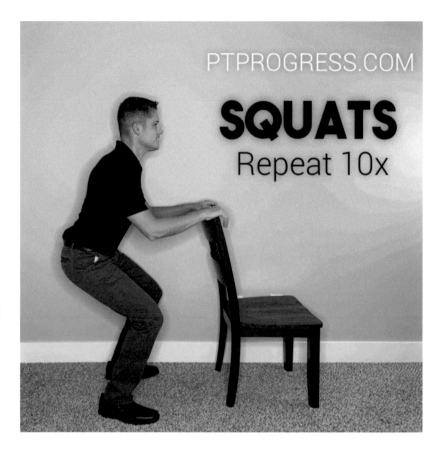

*If you've ever felt unstable when sitting or standing up from a chair,  this is a great exercise to build strength and coordination!*

# Tandem Stance or Semi-Tandem

**Instructions:**

*Stand with one foot in front of the other so you are in a 'heel-toe' position.*

*If this is too difficult initially, move your feet apart slightly. Use a counter or chair as support if you need.*

**Hold this position for 10 seconds on each side. Repeat 2 to 3 times.**

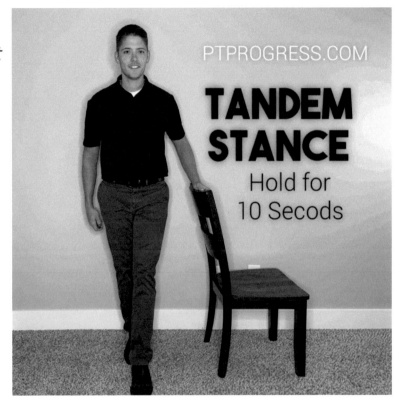

*This balance exercise is great to practice because it puts your body into a narrow stance. With a decreased base of support, you are challenging your muscles to keep you centered!*

# Heel Raises

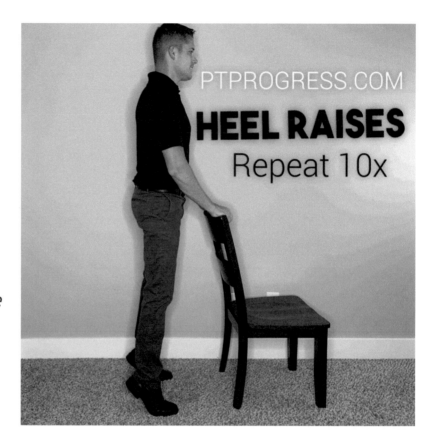

**Instructions:**

Stand with your feet shoulder width apart. While holding onto a counter or firm surface, lift your heels off the ground. You should feel most of the pressure on the front of your feet like you're standing on your toe.

It's ok to put pressure into the counter with your hands at first.

Make sure you stay tall and avoid leaning. Progress this exercise by applying less pressure with your arms and eventually performing without holding counter.

**Perform 10 repetitions.**
**Repeat 2 to 3 times.**

Calf strength is important for balance because this muscle controls our ankle position. When we feel unsteady or need to correct our balance, we use our ankle muscles to reposition our body. Stronger calf muscles can lead to better balance!

# Hamstring Stretch

**Instructions:** *Stand with your leg on a step or on the ground slightly in front of your body. Keep your back straight and gently lean forward feeling a stretch in the back of the thigh and knee.*

*Another way to stretch the hamstring is to sit and extend your leg, leaning forward until you feel a gentle pulling sensation.*

**Hold each stretch for 10 to 20 seconds.**
**Repeat 2 to 3 times on both legs.**

*This is an important exercise for improving balance because the hamstrings can become very tight as we age. This usually happens due to sitting for prolonged periods.*

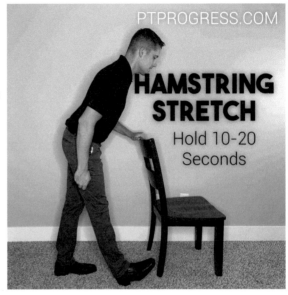

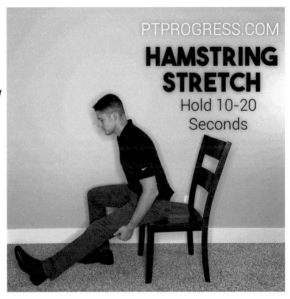

*Improving flexibility in the hamstrings can help to decrease cramping or spasms in the hamstring when you first stand up.*

# Calf Stretch

**Instructions:** *Stand with your foot against a step and gently lean forward while holding onto the railing or a countertop.*

*You should feel a gentle pulling in your calf or ankle as you hold for 10 to 20 seconds. Avoid bouncing or rocking back and forth.*

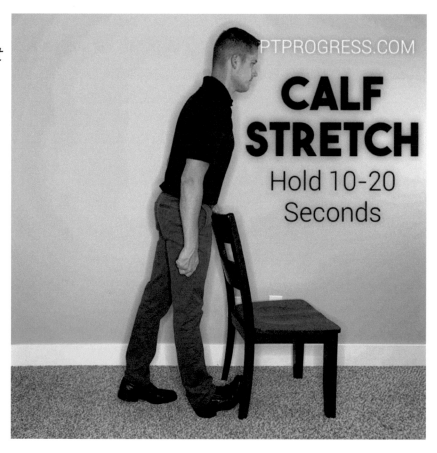

**Hold this stretch for 10 to 20 seconds each leg. Repeat 2 to 3 times.**

*Stretching the calf can help relieve soreness and cramps in the lower leg. If you ever experienced a 'charlie horse' in your leg that almost took you off your feet, this calf stretch is a great exercise to perform!*

# APPENDIX

# Appendix A

## Balancing Act Exercise Diary

Instructions:
- Fill in the number of the exercise you are doing (1-20)
- Follow the instructions for each exercise
- Record in the Exercise Diary how many seconds you were able to hold the exercise (Time) and the hand position (HP) you used
- Track your progress over the days, trying to improve your time and difficulty
- You can keep additional notes as to whether your eyes were open or closed

*See Example of Exercise Diary on page 24*

# Balancing Act Exercise Diary

NAME: _____

Fill in the Exercise # you are doing. Each time you do the exercise record how many seconds you held the exercise (Time) and the hand position (HP) you used.

| Week 1 | Exercise # | | Exercise # | | Exercise # | | Exercise # | | Exercise # | |
|---|---|---|---|---|---|---|---|---|---|---|
| | Time | HP | Time | HP | Time | HP | Time | HP | Time | HP |
| Day1 | | | | | | | | | | |
| Day 2 | | | | | | | | | | |
| Day 3 | | | | | | | | | | |

| Week 2 | Exercise # | | Exercise # | | Exercise # | | Exercise # | | Exercise # | |
|---|---|---|---|---|---|---|---|---|---|---|
| | Time | HP | Time | HP | Time | HP | Time | HP | Time | HP |
| Day1 | | | | | | | | | | |
| Day 2 | | | | | | | | | | |
| Day 3 | | | | | | | | | | |

| Week 3 | Exercise # | | Exercise # | | Exercise # | | Exercise # | | Exercise # | |
|---|---|---|---|---|---|---|---|---|---|---|
| | Time | HP | Time | HP | Time | HP | Time | HP | Time | HP |
| Day1 | | | | | | | | | | |
| Day 2 | | | | | | | | | | |
| Day 3 | | | | | | | | | | |

| Week 4 | Exercise # | | Exercise # | | Exercise # | | Exercise # | | Exercise # | |
|---|---|---|---|---|---|---|---|---|---|---|
| | Time | HP | Time | HP | Time | HP | Time | HP | Time | HP |
| Day1 | | | | | | | | | | |
| Day 2 | | | | | | | | | | |
| Day 3 | | | | | | | | | | |

# Balancing Act Exercise Diary

NAME: _____

Fill in the Exercise # you are doing. Each time you do the exercise record how many seconds you held the exercise (Time) and the hand position (HP) you used.

| Week 5 | Exercise # | | Exercise # | | Exercise # | | Exercise # | | Exercise # | |
|---|---|---|---|---|---|---|---|---|---|---|
| | Time | HP | Time | HP | Time | HP | Time | HP | Time | HP |
| Day1 | | | | | | | | | | |
| Day 2 | | | | | | | | | | |
| Day 3 | | | | | | | | | | |

| Week 6 | Exercise # | | Exercise # | | Exercise # | | Exercise # | | Exercise # | |
|---|---|---|---|---|---|---|---|---|---|---|
| | Time | HP | Time | HP | Time | HP | Time | HP | Time | HP |
| Day1 | | | | | | | | | | |
| Day 2 | | | | | | | | | | |
| Day 3 | | | | | | | | | | |

| Week 7 | Exercise # | | Exercise # | | Exercise # | | Exercise # | | Exercise # | |
|---|---|---|---|---|---|---|---|---|---|---|
| | Time | HP | Time | HP | Time | HP | Time | HP | Time | HP |
| Day1 | | | | | | | | | | |
| Day 2 | | | | | | | | | | |
| Day 3 | | | | | | | | | | |

| Week 8 | Exercise # | | Exercise # | | Exercise # | | Exercise # | | Exercise # | |
|---|---|---|---|---|---|---|---|---|---|---|
| | Time | HP | Time | HP | Time | HP | Time | HP | Time | HP |
| Day1 | | | | | | | | | | |
| Day 2 | | | | | | | | | | |
| Day 3 | | | | | | | | | | |

# Balancing Act Exercise Diary

NAME: ___*Example*___

Fill in the Exercise # you are doing. Each time you do the exercise record how many seconds you held the exercise (Time) and the hand position (HP) you used.

| Week 1 | Exercise #1 | | Exercise #2 | | Exercise #3 | | Exercise #4 | | Exercise #5 | |
|---|---|---|---|---|---|---|---|---|---|---|
| | Time | HP | Time | HP | Time | HP | Time | HP | Time | HP |
| Day 1 | 20 | 3 | 20 | 3 | 15 | 2/3 | 15 | 1 | 20 | 2/3 |
| Day 2 | 25 | 3 | 22 | 3 | 14 | 2/3 | 13 | 2 | 20 | 3 |
| Day 3 | 30 | 3 | 27 | 3 | 18 | 3 | 20 | 2 | 23 | 3 |
| Week 2 | Exercise #1 | | Exercise #2 | | Exercise #3 | | Exercise #4 | | Exercise #5 | |
| | Time | HP | Time | HP | Time | HP | Time | HP | Time | HP |
| Day 1 | 30 | 2 | 30 | 3 | 18 | 3 | 26 | 2 | 27 | 3 |
| Day 2 | 30 | 3 | 30 | 3 | 25 | 3 | 26 | 3 | 30 | 3 |
| Day 3 | 30 | 3 | 30 | 3 | 30 | 3 | 30 | 3 | 30 | 3 |
| Week 3 | Exercise #6 | | Exercise #7 | | Exercise #8 | | Exercise #9 | | Exercise #10 | |
| | Time | HP | Time | HP | Time | HP | Time | HP | Time | HP |
| Day 1 | 30 | 3 | 15 | 1 | 17 | 1 | 30 | 1 | 19 | 2 |
| Day 2 | 30 | 3 | 15 | 1 | 16 | 2 | 21 | 2 | 21 | 2 |
| Day 3 | | | | | | | | | | |
| Week 4 | Exercise # | | Exercise # | | Exercise # | | Exercise # | | Exercise # | |
| | Time | HP | Time | HP | Time | HP | Time | HP | Time | HP |
| Day 1 | | | | | | | | | | |
| Day 2 | | | | | | | | | | |
| Day 3 | | | | | | | | | | |

# Appendix B

## Social Support Identifier

**Instructions:**
The questions on the next page ask about people in your life who provide you with help or support. For each question list all the people you know, excluding yourself, whom you can count on for help or support in the manner described. Write the person's initials (or name) and their relationship to you (see example). List only one person next to each number for every question.

**Example 1:**

Who do you know you can trust with information that could get you in trouble?

☐ No one

| | | |
|---|---|---|
| 1) T.N. (brother) | 4) Tony (neighbor) | 7) |
| 2) L.M. (friend) | 5) L.M. (employer) | 8) |
| 3) R.S. (friend) | 6) | 9) |

**Example 2:**

Who do you know you can trust with information that could get you in trouble?

☑ No one

| | | |
|---|---|---|
| 1) | 4) | 7) |
| 2) | 5) | 8) |
| 3) | 6) | 9) |

Adapted from: Sarason, I.G., Sarason, B.R.., Shearin, E.N., & Pierce, G.R. (1987). A brief measure of social support: Practical and theoretical implications. *Journal of Social and Personal Relationships, 4*, 497-510.
(Adapted for   Balancing Act Use)

# Social Support Identifier

Please answer all questions as best you can.

**1. Who can you really count on to be dependable when you need help?**

| | | | |
|---|---|---|---|
| 1) | 4) | 7) | ☐ No one |
| 2) | 5) | 8) | |
| 3) | 6) | 9) | |

**2. Who can you really count on to help you feel more relaxed when you are under pressure or tense?**

| | | | |
|---|---|---|---|
| 1) | 4) | 7) | ☐ No one |
| 2) | 5) | 8) | |
| 3) | 6) | 9) | |

**3. Who accepts you totally, including both your worst and your best points?**

| | | | |
|---|---|---|---|
| 1) | 4) | 7) | ☐ No one |
| 2) | 5) | 8) | |
| 3) | 6) | 9) | |

**4. Who do you talk with most frequently either by phone or in person?**

| | | | |
|---|---|---|---|
| 1) | 4) | 7) | ☐ No one |
| 2) | 5) | 8) | |
| 3) | 6) | 9) | |

**5. If you do not feel well, who can you really count on to check in on you and assist you if you need help?**

| | | | |
|---|---|---|---|
| 1) | 4) | 7) | ☐ No one |
| 2) | 5) | 8) | |
| 3) | 6) | 9) | |

**6. If you travel or will be away from home, who can you count on to water your plants, check your mail, take care of your pet, or check on your home?**

| | | | |
|---|---|---|---|
| 1) | 4) | 7) | ☐ No one |
| 2) | 5) | 8) | |
| 3) | 6) | 9) | |

**Social Support Identifier Outcome:**

1. Review answers above. Do any names appear multiple times?
2. For the name that appears frequently, please consider asking this person to support you by calling or stopping by a few times a week to ask how you are doing with your   Balancing Act exercises.
3. If you do not have one name that you wrote in repeatedly, then refer to your answers on Question 4 to identify a support person.

# Appendix C

## Balancing Act

### Description

   Balancing Act is an individual and/or group balance enhancement program designed for anyone who would like to improve his/her balance and reduce the threat of *falls* (see **Appendix E**). There are four levels of exercises: Beginner, Intermediate, Advanced and Action; each with a variety of exercises and additional challenges to master as balance improves. Aside from individual use this program can be prescribed by health care providers and offered by community agencies and organizations (see **Appendix D**).

### Brief History

   Balancing Act was designed in 2010. Our program has been tested with older adults and studies are being expanded to measure more factors that are related to balance and stability when standing and walking. In 2012-13 Balancing Act was awarded the Maine Governor's Award for Fitness Programs in the Special Populations Category.

   In 2013 the National Institutes of Health awarded $380,000 to researchers at the University of New England (UNE) College of Osteopathic Medicine (COM), University of Maine Center on Aging, and The Iris Network to study a falls prevention program for older citizens with vision impairment. The Balancing Act Manual was adapted into large print font, audio, and Braille for this study. The outcomes from this grant should be available during 2015-16.

### Falls and How Balancing Act Can Help

   Fatal injuries related to falls are the fifth leading cause of death among older adults in the United States and the second leading cause of death due to associated injuries, and the rates of fall-related deaths are increasing. Each year, falls occur in over a third of persons over age 62, and in over half of persons over age 75. A substantial proportion of these falls are preventable, an important risk factor that can be changed is poor balance. Falling doesn't have to be a part of the aging process. Fear of falling can increase your fall risk, especially when it is combined with decreased activity levels.

   The Balancing Act exercise program provides you with an opportunity to practice and improve your balance in a safe and controlled environment. Setting aside time each day to practice these exercises will improve your overall balance ability during daily tasks.

### Benefits of Balance Training

   Performing balance exercises 3-5 days per week can provide tremendous benefits, such as:

- Increases joint stability, muscle strength, muscle mass, and flexibility
- Improves muscle endurance
- Increases performance for all physical activity
- Stimulates brain activity
- Reduces serious injury should a fall occur

# Appendix D

## Key Points for Health Providers and Community Organizations

**Healthcare Providers**

The Balancing Act program can be prescribed for your patients to help improve balance, reduce the risk of falling, and the fear of falling. Once you have established that your patient is at risk for falls, there are two avenues you can take with this manual: (1) hand the patient the manual and ask her/him to start with beginner exercises; or (2) perform either the Tinetti Gait and Balance test OR the Timed Get up and Go test to determine the starting level for the Balancing Act program.

- Beginner Level – **Tinetti Score** ≤19 – **Get up and Go time** $\geq$ 20 seconds
- Intermediate Level – **Tinetti Score** 19-23 – **Get up and Go time** 12-19 seconds
- Advanced Level – **Tinetti Score** ≥24 – **Get up and Go time** $\leq$ 11 seconds

The recommended prescription for this program is to exercise 3-4 days per week for a total of fifteen minutes per day, performing the 5 exercises in a given level (i.e. Beginner) Help set goals with your patients. For example, encourage your patients to keep track of their progress with the Exercise Diary in **Appendix A** and suggest they fill out the Social Support Identifier in **Appendix B** to help with reminders to do the exercises.

**Community Agencies and Organizations**

Balancing Act is easily implemented in small groups either utilizing the lay leader model or staff leadership. For community agencies and organizations that want to offer Balancing Act, we can provide employees with Balancing Act training to familiarize staff with the programs details. These trainings can be very useful to ensure that the program is maximizing it's full potential and can be a great gateway for future programs. During these trainings, staff asks for feedback from community organizations so as to continue adapting the program for older adults.

If your community agency or organization is interested in having staff come to your site for a hands on training please contact us (contact information can be found on page i).

Community agencies and organizations can use the Balancing Act program in group classes or for individual use. Suggestions and tips for either use are listed next: 1. Group Classes & 2. Individual Users.

### 1. Group Classes

The Balancing Act program can be used as the focus for small group sessions or can be included as a component of a group class. If you have a group of people interested in participating in the Balancing Act exercises, this manual can be used as a guideline for those group sessions. When planning to start a Balancing Act Group class the following considerations should be made:

- Provide a safe classroom environment (even floors, enough space, emergency procedures) with plenty of stable objects to provide hand support.
- Form groups of participants with similar balance abilities – this helps the instructor provide directions appropriate for all participants.
- Group class size depends on the room size and the ability of the instructor. Groups of 4-8 people are a very manageable size.

During the first group class is it important to make sure all instructors and participants are comfortable with the material and the goals of the program. We suggest groups start at the beginning of the manual, and to verbalize the following:

- Hand Positions
- Start Position
- How to make exercises more challenging (reducing contact with hands, closing eyes, etc)

Once the balance ability of all participants has been gauged class leaders can increase difficulty by progressing through the challenges and exercise levels based on participants' abilities. Increases in difficulty should be done on an individual basis, when participants feel comfortable doing the previous exercise without holding on. Encourage participants to challenge themselves, working through the stages of hand positions, proper body positions, and making each exercise a bit harder by adding the challenges listed under "Too Easy?" at the end of each exercise.

### 2. Individual Users

The Balancing Act Manual can be handed out to members of community centers, senior centers, churches, Area Agencies on Aging, etc. If centers choose not to run group classes, individuals can use the manual independently (details provided on page 2 – Getting Started). Centers and organizations can register participants at their sites and provide extra support by calling the participants once a week to check on progress or have the participants submit their Balancing Act Exercise Diary (see **Appendix A**) once a week or month, whichever works for the center.

Participants should progress on their own based on how balanced they feel. However, if it is noticed that a person continues to do beginner exercises and is not advancing this could be a sign that they may not be practicing enough or may not understand how to progress to the next exercise level. Review the Checklist at the end of each exercise level (Beginner, Intermediate, and Advanced) with the participant to determine his/her ability.

# Appendix E

## Glossary

**Balance:** even distribution of weight enabling someone to remain upright and steady.

**Base of Support:** the location on the body where most of the weight is supported; the legs and feet make up the body's base of support, acting as the base or foundation to standing erect so as to keep from falling, sinking, or slipping.

**Center of Gravity:** the point at which the entire weight of a body is concentrated so that at this point the body maintains its equilibrium (balance) in any position.

**Fall:** coming to rest inadvertently on the ground or at a lower level.

**Points of Contact:** the area in contact with the floor or another stable object (feet, hands holding on, touch with finger tips).

**Postural Sway:** the body sway induced by performing balance exercises. To sway is to move rhythmically back and forth or to influence body position.

**Proprioception:** the ability to sense the position, location, orientation, and movement of one's body.

**Stability:** the state or quality of being stable (firmness of position), especially being resistant to change.

**Social Support:** is the existence of people on whom we can rely and will provide assistance. They are the ones who let us know that they care about, value and respect us. Support can come from many sources, such as family, friends, coworkers, etc.

**Vestibular/Vestibular System:** the system in the human body that contributes to balance and to the sense of where the body is in relation to its surroundings. It is the sensory system that gives feedback about movement and sense of balance.

**Visual Point of Reference:** a constant visual cue or focal point that the eyes concentrate on to aid balance and stability; best visual points of reference are at eye level when standing tall.

# Appendix F

## Information
## _ [Exercise and Conditioning for Easier Living]

### Description
is a community-based comprehensive health promotion program created to serve older adults living independently or in long term care environments.  provides an array of programs focused on balance, falls prevention, physical activity and wellness. Programs are designed to be provided in a group or individual format.

### Mission
U-ExCEL's mission is to optimize the health and well-being of older adults through fitness and wellness programming.

### Program Offerings
is constantly expanding its program offerings to meet the needs of older adults living in a variety of community environments. A sample of our programs include:

- **Balancing Act:** See **Appendix C**.
- **Education Series**: This program series allows for  staff to provide an educational program to participants on a variety of health related topics. Examples include: "The Importance of Play"; "Beating the Winter Blues"; "Take 5 Minutes to Improve Your Health"; etc.
- **Movement to Music:** This movement based class is designed to keep you moving (exercising) to different music during the class whether you know how to dance or not.  Anyone can join regardless of ability.
- **Range of Motion:**  This slow paced class focuses on emphasizing and maximizing the movements in all joints; beginning with the head, working out to the fingers, and down to the toes. Individuals can sit or stand to participate in this class. There are no weights used and participants do not have to get down on the floor.
- **Sit and Fit:** This unique class includes chair exercises that promote flexibility, cardiovascular fitness, dexterity, and fun. It is amazing how much exercising can be done in a chair.
  - **Modified Sit and Fit:** Same as Sit and Fit but includes higher level exercises that are done while standing behind the chair.
- **Strength and Balance:** This class is designed to improve functional ability by strengthening the muscles and improving static and dynamic balance.
- **Water Aerobics:** Fun and energizing exercises done in the water that include a combination of cardiovascular, range of motion, flexibility, and muscular strength exercises.
- **Water Walking:** A half-hour of creative and dynamic ways to walk in the water, which is equivalent to one hour of walking on land.
- **Yog-Chi:** This unique slower-paced class will combine principles from yoga and Tai-Chi, be slow paced, and will continue to adapt, incorporating additional techniques, poses, and so on as the class and instruction evolves.

Made in United States
Troutdale, OR
01/02/2024

16598733R00033